Cambridge Elements ≡

Elements in High-Risk Pregnancy: Management Options
edited by
David James
University of Nottingham
Philip Steer
Imperial College London
Carl Weiner
Creighton University School of Medicine
Stephen Robson
Newcastle University

CAESAREAN SECTION DELIVERY

Joshua D. Dahlke
Nebraska Methodist Hospital and Perinatal Center
Suneet P. Chauhan
Delaware Center for Maternal and Fetal Medicine of Christiana Care Inc.

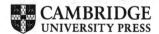

CAMBRIDGE
UNIVERSITY PRESS

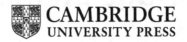

Shaftesbury Road, Cambridge CB2 8EA, United Kingdom

One Liberty Plaza, 20th Floor, New York, NY 10006, USA

477 Williamstown Road, Port Melbourne, VIC 3207, Australia

314–321, 3rd Floor, Plot 3, Splendor Forum, Jasola District Centre,
New Delhi – 110025, India

103 Penang Road, #05–06/07, Visioncrest Commercial, Singapore 238467

Cambridge University Press is part of Cambridge University Press & Assessment,
a department of the University of Cambridge.

We share the University's mission to contribute to society through the pursuit of
education, learning and research at the highest international levels of excellence.

www.cambridge.org
Information on this title: www.cambridge.org/9781009479479

DOI: 10.1017/9781009479493

When citing this work, please include a reference to the DOI 10.1017/9781009479493

First published 2025

A catalogue record for this publication is available from the British Library

ISBN 978-1-009-47947-9 Paperback
ISSN 2976-8330 (online)
ISSN 2976-8322 (print)

Cambridge University Press & Assessment has no responsibility for the persistence
or accuracy of URLs for external or third-party internet websites referred to in this
publication and does not guarantee that any content on such websites is, or will
remain, accurate or appropriate.

Every effort has been made in preparing this Element to provide accurate and
up-to-date information which is in accord with accepted standards and practice at the
time of publication. Although case histories are drawn from actual cases, every effort
has been made to disguise the identities of the individuals involved. Nevertheless, the
authors, editors and publishers can make no warranties that the information
contained herein is totally free from error, not least because clinical standards are
constantly changing through research and regulation. The authors, editors and
publishers therefore disclaim all liability for direct or consequential damages resulting
from the use of material contained in this Element. Readers are strongly advised to pay
careful attention to information provided by the manufacturer of any drugs or
equipment that they plan to use.

Caesarean Section Delivery

Elements in High-Risk Pregnancy: Management Options

DOI: 10.1017/9781009479493
First published online: January 2025

Joshua D. Dahlke
Nebraska Methodist Hospital and Perinatal Center

Suneet P. Chauhan
Delaware Center for Maternal and Fetal Medicine of Christiana Care Inc.

Author for correspondence: Joshua D. Dahlke, joshuadahlke@gmail.com

Abstract: Caesarean section delivery (CD) is the most common surgical operation performed in the world. Since first described 400 years ago, surgical rates continue to rise globally. Caesarean rates are now reported from South American countries of over 50% and rates of over 32% are currently being reported from the United States, China, England and Scotland. Surgical complications can occur at the time of operation and there are major implications for future pregnancies, including increased rates of placenta previa/accreta, stillbirth and preterm labour. This Element discusses many aspects of CD, including the Robson 10 group classification system, which classifies populations by characteristics such as parity, presentation of the fetus and the history of previous births, an evidence-based approach to surgical techniques, recommendations of the major guidelines and recommendations concerning trial of labour after previous caesarean.

Keywords: caesarean, Robson criteria, surgery, surgical technique, trial of labour after caesarean

ISBNs: 9781009479479 (PB), 9781009479493 (OC)
ISSNs: 2976-8330 (online), 2976-8322 (print)

Contents

1 Commentary

Caesarean section delivery (CD) is the most common surgical operation performed in the world. Although successful caesareans (in which the mother and baby survived) were reported more than 400 years ago, it was not until the development of safe anaesthetics, blood transfusion, antibiotics and improved surgical techniques in the first half of the twentieth century that the rates started to rise globally. The evidence suggests that CD rates of 10–15% reduce maternal and perinatal mortality. Although there are still many parts of the world where a minimum safe number of caesareans are still not available, CD rates have generally burgeoned such that rates of over 50% are now reported from South American countries such as Chile, Argentina and Brazil, and rates of over 32% are currently being reported from the United States, China, England and Scotland. This raises the question as to whether too many caesareans are being done. Not only can there be surgical complications for the mother at the time of operation and in the puerperium, there are major implications for future pregnancies, including increased rates of placenta previa/accreta, stillbirth and preterm labour. Thus, the number of future pregnancies the mother plans should be taken into account when deciding to recommend a CD. Moreover, abdominal delivery of the baby prevents it acquiring the mother's gastrointestinal microbiome, a process that occurs naturally during vaginal birth, and the consequences may include associated increased rates of allergy and obesity.

Attempts to restrict caesarean section rates to those that are medically justified have been largely unsuccessful. Part of the problem is establishing rates that are appropriate for a particular population. One approach has been to use the Robson 10 group classification system (TGCS), which classifies populations by characteristics such as parity, presentation of the fetus and the history of previous births. In many studies, up to a third of caesareans are carried out simply because the previous delivery was also a caesarean, and so the indications for a primary (first) caesarean section must always be evaluated particularly carefully. Whenever a caesarean section is performed, it is vital that appropriate surgical techniques are used. In this Element we summarise the recommendations of the major guidelines. We also summarise the recommendations concerning trial of labour after previous caesarean.

2 Introduction

Caesarean rates vary across countries, ranging from over 50% in South American countries such as Chile, Argentina and Brazil to over 32% in the United States and China.[1–5] Approximately 1.1 million caesareans are performed in the United States and almost 30 million neonates are born worldwide via caesarean on an annual basis.[6,7] In general, maternal morbidity and mortality among women who undergo CD remains substantially higher compared with women who deliver vaginally, and these risks increase with each subsequent caesarean.[8,9] Moreover, given the multifactorial nature of indications, the optimal caesarean rate is difficult to determine. As such, national goals to reduce the caesarean rate, such as the Healthy People campaign in the United States, have had to be adapted due to an inability to reduce the incidence of this common surgery.[10,11,12] A particular reason to limit the use of caesarean section has been the growing understanding that as well as CD being associated with higher rates of short-term neonatal morbidity such as transient tachypnea of the newborn (due to retained lung fluid) and respiratory distress syndrome (due to surfactant deficiency),[13] when compared to vaginal birth, infants delivered by caesarean have a 20% increase in the odds of developing asthma and type 1 diabetes in childhood or adulthood.[14,15] Recent studies suggest that these long-term effects may be due to marked differences in the gut microbiome between neonates born by CD who acquire it nosocomially and those delivered vaginally, who have a much greater chance of acquiring the mother's bacteria (which are likely a better match to their genome and to the maternal antibodies present in the newborn's bloodstream).[16]

3 History of CD

The delivery of a fetus surgically through the abdominal wall has a long history. Self-performed caesareans have been described, as have caesareans performed by laypersons, most often in desperation as a result of prolonged labour. However, it was nearly 450 years ago when someone first considered carrying out a caesarean prophylactically in an individual who was unlikely to deliver vaginally and so moribund that death was inevitable. This operative intervention was first described by the French physician François Rousset in 1581. At the time, there was wide criticism from the medical establishment of the day. This was the start of a caesarean debate that continues today, and still with very polarised views. The concept of a risk–benefit ratio has always dominated the discussion, but the nature of the risks and benefits for and against caesarean section have radically changed over time.

During the sixteenth to eighteenth centuries, CD continued to be described, but it remained rare, with most physicians strongly against carrying out the procedure because of its high associated mortality. This mortality was largely related to the poor general condition of the patient at the time the caesarean was carried out, often the result of prolonged labour. This contributed significantly to the risks of infection and haemorrhage as a result of the operation.

In the nineteenth century, an improvement in basic surgical principles and techniques, such as suturing the uterus and employing methods to exteriorise drainage of sepsis and bleeding, helped control the risk of infection and haemorrhage, but caesarean remained an operation that was carried out in extreme circumstances only. The vertical uterine incision remained the most common incision, although Kehrer first described the transverse lower uterine segment caesarean in 1881.[17]

A big advance at the end of the nineteenth century was the use of a tourniquet applied around the lower part of the uterus after the baby had been delivered. This restricted the blood loss while the uterus was being sutured. It was first advocated by Murdoch Cameron (1847–1930) who was Regius Professor of Obstetrics and Gynaecology at the University of Glasgow from 1894 to 1926. He was an advocate of the antiseptic approach of Joseph Lister (1827–1912) and in addition selected his patients by avoiding those whose conditions were already compromised by exhaustion and the infection associated with a long and obstructed labour (his first three caesareans were on rachitic dwarfs who were deemed unable to give birth normally). Cameron's results were very good at the time, relatively speaking, and represented significant progress in the development of the operation. Munro Kerr, a pupil of Cameron's and also from Glasgow, was responsible at the beginning of the twentieth century for developing and encouraging the use of the transverse lower uterine segment incision, publishing his results in 1930.

Although caesarean surgical technique has continued to be debated and improved since the operation was first described, there is little doubt that the greatest advances in the last few years have come with improvement in perioperative care. In particular, improvements in anaesthetic technique have led to more caesareans being performed under regional anaesthesia (epidural or spinal), while the availability of antibiotics and access to blood transfusion have made it much safer.

Caesarean delivery and the optimal rate for this intervention remains controversial, with the pendulum swinging from maybe *too few and too late* to *too many and too early* in many resource-rich countries.[11] Ironically, the controversy in modern obstetrics is the result of the overall success of the procedure. As with other surgical procedures, the safer they become, especially in the short term, the more frequently they are performed. This could be considered an appropriate clinical response to an altered risk–benefit ratio, but there may always be unforeseen future consequences that may be beneficial or harmful. At the same time, in certain low-resource countries there is still poor access to the operation and insufficient resources to carry it out safely.

4 Primary CD

4.1 Risks (Maternal/Fetal/Neonatal)

Like any other major operation, CD is associated with short-term and long-term complications for the woman and the neonate. The National Institute for Health and Care Excellence guidance on caesarean section initially published in 2011 and updated in 2021 reviewed these risks in detail.[2] The data came from a series of international peer-reviewed studies published between 1996 and 2019. The evidence was categorised into three groups:

- A: Studies that compared outcomes according to the planned mode of delivery (vaginal birth or caesarean section)
- B: Studies that compared outcomes according to the actual mode of delivery but excluding cases of unplanned caesarean section
- C: Studies that compared outcomes according to the actual mode of delivery including both planned and unplanned caesarean section

The risks for women are described in Tables 1 and 3 and those for the baby are described in Table 2.

Outcomes for which there was no evidence of a difference between caesarean and vaginal birth were:

- for women
  - thromboembolic disease
  - major obstetric haemorrhage
  - postnatal depression
  - fecal incontinence more than one year after birth compared with unassisted vaginal delivery
- for babies/children
  - admission to neonatal unit
  - infection
  - persistent verbal delay
  - infant mortality up to one year

Outcomes for which there was conflicting or limited evidence about risk with caesarean or vaginal birth were:

- for women
  - admission to intensive care
  - stillbirth in a subsequent pregnancy

Table 1 Outcomes for women that may be more likely with caesarean birth[2]

Outcomes	Estimated risk with vaginal birth	Calculated risk with caesarean birth	Risk difference	Category of evidence
Peripartum hysterectomy	About 80 women per 100,000 would be expected to have a peripartum hysterectomy (so 99,920 would not)	About 150 women per 100,000 would be expected to have a peripartum hysterectomy (so 99,850 would not)	About 70 more women per 100,000 who had a caesarean birth would be expected to have a peripartum hysterectomy; so for about 99,930 women per 100,000 the outcome was the same irrespective of the method of birth	A – Planned mode of birth
Maternal death	About 4 women per 100,000 would be expected to die (so 99,996 would not)	About 24 women per 100,000 would be expected to die (so 99,976 would not)	About 20 more women per 100,000 who had a caesarean birth would be expected to die; so for about 99,980 women per 100,000 the outcome was the same irrespective of the method of birth	A – Planned mode of birth
Length of hospital stay	About 2 and a half days on average	About 4 days on average	About 1–2 days longer on average for caesarean birth [2011]	A – Planned mode of birth

Table 1 (cont.)

Outcomes	Estimated risk with vaginal birth	Calculated risk with caesarean birth	Risk difference	Category of evidence
Placenta accreta in a future pregnancy	About 40 women per 100,000 would be expected to have a placenta accreta (so 99,960 would not)	About 100 women per 100,000 would be expected to have a placenta accreta (so 99,900 would not)	About 60 more women per 100,000 who had a caesarean birth would be expected to have a placenta accreta; so for about 99,940 women per 100,000 the outcome was the same irrespective of the method of birth	C – Actual mode of birth (including planned and unplanned caesarean)
Uterine rupture in a future pregnancy or birth	About 40 women per 100,000 would be expected to have a uterine rupture in a future pregnancy (so 99,960 would not)	About 1,020 women per 100,000 would be expected to have a uterine rupture in a future pregnancy (so 98,980 would not)	About 960 more women per 100,000 who had a caesarean birth would be expected to have a uterine rupture in a future pregnancy; so for about 99,020 women per 100,000 the outcome was the same irrespective of the method of birth	C – Actual mode of birth (including planned and unplanned caesarean)

Key: The outcomes labelled [2011] are outcomes that were not reviewed in 2021 but the Committee considered were still applicable and were carried forwards.

Table 2 Outcomes for babies that may be more likely with caesarean birth[2]

Outcomes	Estimated risk with vaginal birth	Calculated risk with caesarean birth	Risk difference	Category of evidence
Neonatal mortality	About 30 babies per 100,000 would be expected to die (so 99,970 would not)	About 50 babies per 100,000 would be expected to die (so 98,950 would not)	About 20 more women per 100,000 whose mothers had a caesarean birth would be expected to die; so for about 99,980 babies per 100,000 the outcome was the same irrespective of the method of birth	A – Planned mode of birth
Asthma	About 1,500 per 100,000 children would be expected to have asthma (so 98,500 would not)	About 1,810 per 100,000 children would be expected to have asthma (so 98,190 would not)	About 310 more children per 100,000 whose mothers had a caesarean birth would be expected to have asthma; so for about 99,690 babies or children per 100,000 the outcome was the same irrespective of the method of birth	B – Actual mode of birth (excluding unplanned caesarean)
Childhood obesity	About 4,050 per 100,000 children would be expected to be obese (so 95,950 would not)	About 4,560 children per 100,000 would be expected to be obese (so 95,450 would not)	About 510 children per 100,000 whose mothers who had a caesarean birth would be expected to be obese; so for about 99,490 women per 100,000 the outcome was the same irrespective of the method of birth	B – Actual mode of birth (excluding unplanned caesarean)

Table 3 Outcomes for women that may be less likely with caesarean birth[2]

Outcomes	Estimated risk with vaginal birth	Calculated risk with caesarean birth	Risk difference	Category of evidence
Urinary incontinence occurring more than one year after birth	About 48,700 women per 100,000 would be expected to have urinary incontinence (so 51,300 would not)	About 27,520 women per 100,000 would be expected to have urinary incontinence (so 77,480 would not)	About 21,180 fewer women per 100,000 who had a caesarean birth would be expected to have urinary incontinence; so for about 78,820 women per 100,000 the outcome was the same irrespective of the method of birth	B – Actual mode of birth (excluding unplanned caesarean)
Fecal incontinence occurring more than one year after birth; compared to assisted vaginal birth	About 15,100 women per 100,000 would be expected to have fecal incontinence after an assisted vaginal birth (so 84,900 would not)	About 7,410 women per 100,000 would be expected to have fecal incontinence (so 92, 590 would not)	About 7,690 fewer women per 100,000 who had a caesarean birth would be expected to have fecal incontinence; so for about 92,310 women per 100,000 the outcome was the same irrespective of the method of birth	B – Actual mode of birth (excluding unplanned caesarean)

				A – Planned mode of birth
Vaginal tear: third- and fourth-degree tears	About 560 women per 100,000 would be expected to have a third- or fourth-degree vaginal tear (so 99,400 would not)	About 0 women per 100,000 would be expected to have a third- or fourth-degree vaginal tear (so 100,000 would not)	About 560 fewer women per 100,000 who had a caesarean birth would be expected to have a third- or fourth-degree vaginal tear; so for about 99,440 women per 100,000 the outcome was the same irrespective of the method of birth [2011]	A – Planned mode of birth
Pain during birth, 3 days after birth and 4 months after birth (as measured with the Visual Analogue Scale [VAS]; 0 is no pain, 10 is most severe pain)	Median pain score of 8 (during birth), 4 (3 days after birth) and 0 (4 months after birth)	Median pain score of 1 (during birth), 5 (3 days after birth) and 0 (4 months after birth)	Reduction of pain score with caesarean birth compared with vaginal birth of 7 (during birth), reduction of pain score with vaginal birth compared with caesarean birth of 1 (3 days after birth) and no difference between vaginal birth and caesarean birth (4 months after birth) [2011]	A – Planned mode of birth

Key: The outcomes labelled [2011] are outcomes that were not reviewed in 2021 but the Committee considered were still applicable and were carried forwards.

- for babies/children
  - ○ respiratory morbidity
  - ○ cerebral palsy
  - ○ autism spectrum condition
  - ○ type 1 diabetes

4.2 Management Options: Prenatal

4.2.1 Indications for Caesarean Section

To minimise these complications, it is important to limit the number of caesareans to those with clear indications (which can be medical, psychological, or a fully informed choice by the patient), and at the same time to optimise the methods employed in performing this surgery. Strategies to limit or reduce surgical interventions in general and caesarean rates in particular have generally been unsuccessful for a number of reasons.[10,11,12,18] However, some studies have reported successful strategies that have led to the introduction of the concept of an 'appropriate caesarean rate' where the CD rate is broken down into groups of women with different characteristics (e.g. the Robson 10 groups) and interpreted in relation to maternal and neonatal outcomes.[19, 20]

The Robson 10 group classification system provides one approach to optimise caesarean rate reduction in the context of various clinically relevant stratifications, summarised in Table 4.[21] Simultaneously, additional research has focused on trying to improve and standardise perioperative care, and in particular surgical techniques to ensure that each caesarean is performed according to the best evidence available.[20,21]

Table 4 TGCS for caesarean deliveries[21]

Group	Description	Proportion of total deliveries (%)	Caesarean rate in group (%)
1	Nulliparous, single cephalic, ≥37 weeks, spontaneous labour	23.3	7.1
2	Nulliparous, single cephalic, ≥37 weeks, induced or caesarean before labour	14.9	35.9
3	Multiparous (excluding previous caesareans), single cephalic, ≥37 weeks, spontaneous labour	29.3	1.2

Table 4 (cont.)

Group	Description	Proportion of total deliveries (%)	Caesarean rate in group (%)
4	Multiparous (excluding previous caesareans), single cephalic, ≥37 weeks, induced or caesarean before labour	10.8	13.8
5	Previous caesarean, single cephalic, ≥37 weeks	11.5	68.1
6	All nulliparous breeches	2.0	93.8
7	All multiparous breeches (including previous caesareans)	1.6	89.9
8	All multiple pregnancies (including previous caesareans)	2.3	65.7
9	All abnormal lies (including previous caesareans)	0.5	100.0
10	All single cephalic, <37 weeks (including previous caesareans)	3.9	30.4

Prevalence of specific groups derived from the National Maternity Hospital, Ireland in 2013[22]

Auditing the indications for caesarean remains difficult as the indications vary between studies, are difficult to define, inconsistently used, often multiple, and sometimes not recorded at all. A retrospective cohort trial of over 38,000 primary caesareans among over 228,000 deliveries at participating sites carried out in the United States by the Consortium for Safe Labor suggests that if the results are nationally representative, approximately 70% of caesareans performed in the United States are primary (first) births and repeat caesarean accounts for 30% of the total caesarean rate.[23]

Table 5 summarises the most common indications for primary caesarean in this large cohort. Notably, intrapartum arrest disorders (arrest of dilation, arrest of descent), suspected fetal compromise (non-reassuring fetal status), and malpresentation accounted for almost 80% of the indications for primary caesarean. Less common indications include multiple gestation, suspected macrosomia, maternal HIV or herpes simplex virus (HSV), pre-eclampsia, non-medically indicated (maternal request), or other factors (uterine rupture, cord prolapse, placenta or vasa previa, abruption, or other obstetric emergency). Furthermore, in those with

Table 5 Indications for primary caesarean[23]

Indications for primary caesarean	Total	Primiparous	Multiparous
Fetal			
Malpresentation (breech)	18.5	16.0	26.0
Multiple gestation	3.0	2.5	5.0
Suspected macrosomia	3.0	3.0	3.7
Maternal			
Infectious vertical transmission risk (HIV, HSV)	1.0	1.0	1.5
Obstetric factors (uterine rupture, cord prolapse, placenta or vasa previa, abruption, or other obstetric emergency)	2.5	2.0	5.5
History of uterine surgery	2.0	1.5	4.0
Repeat			
Maternal request (non-medically indicated)	3.0	3.0	3.0
Pre-eclampsia	3.5	3.5	3.0
Other (not otherwise specified)	9.0	8.5	10.5
Intrapartum			
Suspected fetal compromise	24.0	23.0	25.0
Arrest disorders (dilation, descent)	35.0	41.0	19.5

a history of prior caesarean, over 80% are delivered via repeat caesarean in subsequent pregnancies.[23] The approach to optimising management of those with a prior caesarean is further discussed in Section 5.

4.2.2 Primary Prevention of the First CD

A discussion of delivery following caesarean cannot be complete without mentioning the evidence base for primary prevention of the first caesarean. Recent joint efforts by the American College of Obstetricians and Gynecologists (ACOG) and the Society for Maternal–Fetal Medicine (SMFM) have endorsed the promotion of evidence-based approaches to preventing primary caesarean. Table 6 summarises these recommendations.[24] By more clearly defining latent and active phases of labour, establishing stricter criteria for arrest disorders, and prioritising interventions such as amnioinfusion, manual rotation, scalp stimulation, and operative

Table 6 Recommendations for safe prevention of primary caesarean

Factor	Recommendation
General/prenatal	Individuals, organisations, and governing bodies should work to ensure that research conducted provides better knowledge to guide decisions regarding CS and encourage policy changes that safely lower the rate of primary CS
	Women should be counseled about Institute of Medicine (IOM) maternal weight guidelines in an attempt to avoid excessive weight gain
	Fetal presentation should be assessed and documented beginning at 36^{+0} weeks to allow external cephalic version to be offered
Induction of labour	Before 41^{+0} weeks, induction of labour should be performed based on maternal and fetal indications. Inductions at $\geq 41^{+0}$ weeks of gestation should be performed to reduce risk of CS and risk of perinatal morbidity and mortality
	Cervical ripening methods should be used when labour is induced in women with unfavourable cervix
	CS for failed induction of labour in the latent phase can be avoided by allowing longer durations of the latent phase (up to 24 hours) and requiring that oxytocin be administered for at least 12–18 hours after membrane rupture before deeming induction failure
	CS to avoid potential birth trauma should be limited to estimated fetal weights of at least 5,000 g in women without diabetes and at least 4,500 g in women with diabetes. Birth weight $\geq 5,000$ g is rare, and patients should be counseled that estimates of fetal weight, particularly late in gestation, are imprecise
	Perinatal outcomes when the first twin is in cephalic presentation are not improved by CS. Thus, women with either cephalic/cephalic or cephalic/noncephalic twins should be counseled to attempt vaginal delivery
Progress of labour – first stage	Prolonged latent phase (>20 hours in nulliparous women and >14 hours in parous women) should not be an indication for CS

Table 6 (cont.)

Factor	Recommendation
	Slow but progressive dilatation in the first stage of labour should not be an indication for CS
	Cervical dilatation of 6 cm should be considered the threshold for active phase of most women in labour
	CS for active-phase arrest in the first stage of labour should be reserved for women ≥6 cm of dilatation with ruptured membranes who fail to progress despite four hours of adequate uterine activity, or at least six hours of oxytocin administration with inadequate uterine activity and no cervical change
	A specific absolute maximum length of time spent in second stage of labour beyond which all women should undergo operative delivery has not been identified
	Amnioinfusion for repetitive variable fetal heart rate decelerations may safely reduce the rate of CS
	Scalp stimulation can be used as a means of assessing fetal acid–base status when abnormal or indeterminate (formerly, non-reassuring) fetal heart patterns are present, and is a safe alternative to CS in this setting
Progress of labour – second stage	Before diagnosing arrest of labour in second stage, if maternal and fetal conditions permit, allow for the following: • at least two hours of pushing in parous women • at least three hours of pushing in nulliparous women Longer durations may be appropriate (e.g. with use of epidural analgesia or with fetal malposition) as long as progress is being documented
	Operative vaginal delivery in second stage of labour by experienced and well-trained physicians should be considered a safe, acceptable alternative to CS
	Manual rotation of fetal occiput in setting of fetal malposition in second stage of labour is a reasonable intervention to consider before moving to operative vaginal delivery or CS

Based on ACOG, AMFM. Am J Obstet Gynecol 2014; 210: 179–93[25] vaginal delivery, it is the goal of these organisations to minimise non-indicated primary CS, while achieving the right balance of safe management of labour to minimise maternal and neonatal morbidity.

4.2.3 Counselling Women[2]

All women should be offered the opportunity to discuss the mode of birth early during the pregnancy. The discussion should enable them to make informed decisions about childbirth. Information given should be evidence based and presented in a way that the woman understands, is suitable for her, and takes into account any personal, cultural, or religious factors. The woman's views should be at the core of decisions made.

Information that should be discussed includes:

- explaining that 25–30% of women have a CD
- the accepted indications for the procedure (80% of operations are undertaken for either malpresentations, poor progress in labour, or suspected fetal compromise) (see Table 5 for details)
- what the procedure involves
- what the relative risks are when comparing vaginal birth with a caesarean birth (see Tables 1, 2, and 3) and mention those outcomes for which there seems to be do difference between either mode of birth

4.3 Management Options: Labour/Delivery

4.3.1 Surgical Technique

As previously mentioned, CD is the most commonly performed major abdominal surgery in the world, with almost 30 million neonates delivered by caesarean worldwide in 2015 (see Example of CD www.youtube.com/watch? v=IFU9o0OIcwc&t=875s).[1] In the United states, approximately 1.1 million CDs were performed in 2019.[2] Evidence-based surgical techniques were synthesised in two systematic reviews that summarised 155 randomised clinical trials (RCTs), meta-analyses, or systematic reviews performed from 1960–2012 for each technical aspects of CD.[26, 27] Using identical search criteria as those systematic reviews, Dahlke et al. identified an additional 217 RCTs, meta-analyses, or systematic reviews published from October 2012 through October 2019 addressing at least one aspect of CD surgical technique, and published a commentary to offer an evidence-based, standardised CD surgical technique informed by the 370+ RCTs, meta-analyses, and systematic reviews.[28] The rationale to standardise the surgical technique was based on three arguments: 1) other standardised protocols incorporated within institutions improve safety, efficiency, and effectiveness in healthcare systems; 2) surgical training among those learning the procedure could become consistent and uniform across hospitals and regions; and 3) standardising techniques would strengthen future trials by minimising the potential for aspects of the surgery not being studied to bias results.[28]

The NICE guideline (NG192) on caesarean birth provides a similar evidence-based approach to many of the procedural aspects of the operation.[2] In addition to surgical techniques, it expands recommendations to include when to offer CD as well as postpartum care of the patient after CD. The goals of both the commentary by Dahlke et al. and the NICE guidelines are congruent, with the aim to improve the consistency and quality of care for individuals giving birth via CD.

Table 7 summarises and compares the technical aspects recommended by NICE and Dahlke, and there are notable differences. For example, the NICE guideline

Table 7 Comparison of evidence-based caesarean technique

Caesarean technique	Standardised caesarean[28]	NICE[2]
Prophylactic antibiotics	• Pre-incision ampicillin or first-generation cephalosporin • Add azithromycin 500 mg intravenously (IV) if labour before CD	Pre-incision antibiotics
Thromboprophylaxis	Sequential compression devices prior to surgery	Offer according to risk (graduated stockings, hydration, early mobilisation, low-molecular-weight heparin)
Lateral tilt	Omit	Perform up to 15°
Warming interventions	Standardised maternal active warming interventions	Perform active warming interventions
Supplemental oxygen	Omit	No recommendation
Pre-operative enema	Omit	No recommendation
Skin preparation	Chlorhexidine-alcohol	Chlorhexidine-alcohol

Table 7 (cont.)

Caesarean technique	Standardised caesarean[28]	NICE[2]
Vaginal preparation	Povidone-iodine if labour before CD	Povidone-iodine if labour before CD
Indwelling bladder catheter	Pre-operative placement, removal when feasible post-operatively	Remove no sooner than 12 hours
Incisional adhesive drapes	Omit	No recommendation
Skin, subcutaneous, fascia, and peritoneum entry	Transverse, 2–3 cm above pubic symphysis, sharp subcutaneous and fascia dissection, omit superior and inferior fascia dissection, blunt subcutaneous and fascia expansion, blunt peritoneal entry	Transverse, 2–3 cm above pubic symphysis, sharp subcutaneous and fascia dissection, blunt expansion, blunt peritoneal entry
Barrier retractors	Omit	No recommendation
Bladder flap development	Omit	No recommendation
Uterine incision and expansion	2–3 cm low transverse sharp incision, blunt entry, cephalad-caudad expansion	Blunt entry and expansion
Instrumented delivery	Omit	No recommendation
Uterine atony prevention	Oxytocin 10–40 IU over four to eight hours	Oxytocin 5 IU IV
Placenta removal	Spontaneous	Spontaneous
Intrauterine wiping	Perform only when placental membranes seen	No recommendation
Routine cervical dilation	Omit	No recommendation
Uterine repair: in situ or exteriorised	Exteriorise	In situ

Table 7 (cont.)

Caesarean technique	Standardised caesarean[28]	NICE[2]
Uterine closure	Single layer	Either single or double layer
Elective appendectomy	Omit	No recommendation
Intra-abdominal irrigation	Omit	No recommendation
Peritoneal closure	Omit	Omit
Rectus muscle re-approximation	Omit	No recommendation
Glove change	Omit	Omit
Surgical needle type	Blunt, if available	No recommendation
Fascia closure	Running, with delayed absorbable suture	Running suture
Subcutaneous tissue irrigation	Perform	No recommendation
Subcutaneous tissue closure	Suture closure if ≥2 cm depth	Suture closure if ≥2 cm depth
Skin closure	Subcuticular, absorbable monofilament suture	Suture
Wound dressing	Standard post-surgical wound dressing	No recommendation
Negative pressure wound therapy	Omit	Consider for BMI ≥35

does not offer a recommendation for the following techniques: pre-operative enema, supplemental oxygen use, superior/inferior fascia dissection, bladder flap creation, use of barrier retractors, intra-uterine wiping, routine cervical dilation, intra-abdominal irrigation, and wound dressing. Recommendations that are similar and congruent include pre-incision prophylactic antibiotics (NICE does not include the addition of azithromycin if labour occurs prior to caesarean), thromboprophylaxis, skin and vaginal preparation, indwelling bladder catheter use, abdominal entry technique, blunt uterine incision expansion (NICE does not specify cephalad to caudad expansion), spontaneous placenta removal, oxytocin for atony prevention, running fascia closure, closure of the subcutaneous tissue when ≥2 cm, and skin closure with suture. Specific techniques that differ between the two recommendations include positioning with lateral tilt, in situ versus exteriorisation of the uterus during repair, single- verus double-layer uterine closure, and use of negative pressure wound dressing in those with a body mass index (BMI) >35.

The commentary by Dahlke et al. divided the technical steps in those that could be standardised and incorporated by the surgeon and those that could be standardised and incorporated by institutions after review of the 155 studies from 1960 to 2012 and the additional 216 RCTs, systematic reviews/meta-analyses, and Cochrane reviews completed from 2012 through 2019.[28,29] Notably, more studies on this topic occurred from 2012 to 2019 than the previous 50 years combined. These recommendations and comparison with the NICE guidelines are summarised in Table 7.

4.4 Management Options: Postnatal

4.4.1 Care of the Baby[2]

A paediatrician experienced in neonatal resuscitation should be present for specific deliveries, for example, with a general anaesthetic, the delivery of a preterm baby, or suspected fetal compromise. All babies born by cesearean section are likely to have lower temperature than those born vaginally, so thermal care measures need to be implemented. Women should be offered early 'skin-to-skin' contact with the baby. Women who wish to breast feed their baby should be encouraged and supported to do so as soon as possible after the birth.

4.4.2 Care of the Woman[2]

Following the delivery, a woman should be monitored by appropriately skilled healthcare professionals:

- after a general anaesthetic, for at least two hours until she has airway control, is hemodynamically stable and is able to communicate.
- after a regional anaesthetic (spinal or epidural), until she is hemodynamically stable and has a normal blood pressure. Women who have had diamorphine for the regional block or are at risk of respiratory depression should have the close monitoring continued for at least 12 hours.

Attention should be given to pain management after a caesarean birth. Women with an epidural can be offered intrathecal diamorphine. Other options to be discussed with women include the type of analgesia (which depends on the severity of the pain), the route of administration (oral or injectable either intra-muscularly or intravenously as patient controlled analgesia), and their wish to breast feed. In principle, the aim is to wean women off opioid analgesia as soon as is feasible. The use of opioids may require additional antiemetic medication and laxatives if taken long-term. Oral analgesic agents commonly used are paracetamol and a non-steroidal anti-inflammatory drug (e.g. ibuprofen), provided the latter is not contraindicated. Ideally, these should be given regularly and in combination. If these oral agents do not provide sufficient pain relief, then consideration should be given to adding dihydrocodeine to the paracetamol. However, the latter combination should not be offered to women who are breast feeding because of the risk of neonatal sedation and respiratory depression from the dihydrocodeine. Women can eat and drink normally if they are making an uncomplicated recovery from the operation. There is no evidence that postoperative physiotherapy for women who had a general anaesthetic is of any value.

Women should be advised that their in-hospital stay is likely to be longer than following a vaginal delivery. However, most units now offer discharge after 24 hours with follow-up at home to women who are recovering well and have no problems with their baby. If there are complications in a woman and/or her baby following the delivery, management will need to be customised.

4.4.3 Counselling about Future Pregnancies

Once a woman undergoes a primary caesarean, the mode of delivery in any subsequent pregnancy is affected. For example, the Consortium on Safe Labor in the United States found that a previous uterine scar was the primary indication for over half of all CSs, and that 83% of women with a uterine scar are delivered by CS.[24] The aim of this section is to summarise the best available evidence about risks and benefits associated with delivery in women who have previously undergone CS.

When assessing the evidence on the optimal mode of delivery after previous caesarean, it is important to recognise that much of the data used to counsel women are based on observational trials or expert opinion. While the gold standard to compare outcomes of a trial of labour after caesarean (TOLAC) versus repeat CS would be a well-designed and adequately powered randomised controlled trial (RCT), such a study is unlikely because of the very large numbers that would be required and the fact that most women have a decided view of what they would prefer. A Cochrane review comparing planned repeat CS versus planned vaginal birth in women with a previous caesarean highlighted the paucity of trials that directly assess outcomes between these groups.[30] In this Element, the authors identified two randomised trials involving only 320 women. These two trials had different primary and secondary outcomes, and thus did not provide enough data to definitively recommend one mode of delivery over another with regard to outcomes related to maternal or neonatal morbidity and mortality.

However, many national organisations, including ACOG, the Royal College of Obstetricians and Gynaecologists (RCOG), and the Society of Obstetricians and Gynaecologists of Canada (SOGC), have developed practice guidelines on mode of delivery after previous CS that can assist the provider when discussing the risks and benefits of various aspects of this topic.[24,31,32] While these guidelines incorporate an evidence base for their recommendations, it is notable that variation exists between the three organisations in how the evidence was interpreted and what aspects are highlighted in their respective recommendations, as highlighted in Table 8.

Table 8 Summary of recommendations concerning caesarean and TOLAC from three national guidelines

Clinical factors	Recommendation	National guidelines[a]
Obstetric history		
One low transverse CS	TOLAC recommended	ACOG, RCOG, SOGC
Two low transverse CSs	TOLAC may be considered	ACOG, RCOG
Three or more low transverse CSs	Caesarean recommended	ACOG, RCOG
History of uterine rupture	Caesarean recommended	ACOG, SOGC, RCOG
History of classical scar or scar involving uterine body (e.g. T or J incision)	Caesarean recommended	ACOG, SOGC
History of low vertical uterine incision	TOLAC may be considered	ACOG
Documented details of operative procedure	Not necessary, unless high suspicion of complications	ACOG, SOGC
Current pregnancy		
Twins	TOLAC may be considered	ACOG, RCOG, SOGC
Breech	External cephalic version may be considered	ACOG, SOGC
Diabetes	TOLAC may be considered	SOGC

Table 8 (cont.)

Clinical factors	Recommendation	National guidelines[a]
Preterm birth	TOLAC recommended	RCOG
Prolonged pregnancy (>40 weeks)	TOLAC may be considered	ACOG, SOGC
Short interpregnancy interval (variably defined)	TOLAC may be considered	RCOG, SOGC
Macrosomia	TOLAC may be considered	ACOG, RCOG, SOGC
Delivery location	Hospital only, capable of timely caesarean	ACOG, RCOG, SOGC
Induction of labour		
Overall	Acceptable for maternal or fetal indications	ACOG
	Consultant-led decision	RCOG
Transcervical balloon	Acceptable with prudence	ACOG, SOGC
Oxytocin	Acceptable with prudence	ACOG, SOGC
	Consultant-led decision	RCOG
PGE_2 (dinoprostone)	Not recommended	SOGC
	Consultant-led decision	RCOG
PGE_1 (misoprostol)	Not recommended	ACOG, SOGC
	Consultant-led decision	RCOG
Intrapartum management		
Continuous fetal monitoring	Recommended	ACOG, RCOG, SOGC
Internal tocodynamometry	Routine use not recommended	ACOG, RCOG
Augmentation	Oxytocin acceptable with prudence	ACOG, SOGC
Anaesthesia	Regional analgesia acceptable	ACOG, RCOG

[a] ACOG, American College of Obstetricians and Gynecologists;[24] RCOG, Royal College of Obstetricians and Gynaecologists;[31] SOGC, Society of Obstetricians and Gynaecologists of Canada[32]

4.5 Primary CD: Summary of Management Options

- Prenatal
  - Discuss mode of birth with women early in pregnancy to allow them to make informed choices about childbirth. Important principles are:
    - giving information in a way that the woman understands, taking into account personal, cultural, and religious factors.
    - the woman's view should be central to decision-making.
    - informing women that 25–30% of deliveries are by caesarean.
    - explaining the accepted indications (Table 5).
    - explaining what the procedure involves.
    - discussing the relative risks of vaginal versus caesarean birth (see Tables 1, 2, and 3).
  - Tables 4 and 5 list the indications for the procedure.
  - Implement practices that minimise the likelihood of a CD (see Table 6).
- Labour/delivery
  - Follow evidence-based approaches to all aspects of the procedure (see Table 7).
- Postnatal
  - Care of the baby
    - A paediatrician experienced in neonatal resuscitation should be present for specific deliveries (i.e. use of general anaesthesia, preterm delivery, suspected fetal compromise).
    - Pay attention to thermal care.
    - Encourage early 'skin-to-skin' contact.
    - Offer support women who wish to breast feed.
  - Care of the woman
    - Appropriately skilled healthcare professionals should monitor women postoperatively using guidelines that are dependent on the form of anaesthesia (general or regional).
    - Pain management options include:
      - intrathecal diamorphine whilst an epidural cannula is in place.
      - injectable agents (either intramuscularly or intravenously as patient-controlled analgesia), aiming to wean women off opioid analgesia as soon as is feasible.
      - oral analgesic agents commonly used are paracetamol and a non-steroidal anti-inflammatory drug (provided it is not contraindicated)

given regularly and in combination. If this regimen is inadequate, consider adding dihydrocodeine to the paracetamol, but it is contraindicated in women who are breast feeding.

- Women making an uncomplicated recovery can eat and drink normally.
- Post-operative physiotherapy following a general anaesthetic is of no proven value.

◦ Discuss the implications of the CS for future pregnancies (see Table 8).

5 Secondary/Repeat CD

5.1 Maternal and Neonatal Risks of TOLAC versus Repeat Caesarean

In a systematic review and meta-analysis, Rossi et al. summarised four prospective and three retrospective large cohort studies to determine associated adverse outcomes with four possible scenarios: overall planned TOLAC, successful vaginal birth after caesarean (VBAC), failed TOLAC, and repeat caesarean.[33] In their analysis, maternal and neonatal morbidity such as uterine rupture/dehiscence, blood transfusion, and hysterectomy rates were similar among overall planned TOLAC (including successful VBAC and failed TOLAC) compared to repeat caesarean. Those who experienced a successful VBAC, however, had slightly less maternal morbidity, fewer hysterectomies, and similar uterine rupture/dehiscence and blood transfusion rates compared to scheduled repeat caesarean. In contrast, those who experienced a failed TOLAC had more maternal morbidity, more uterine rupture/dehiscence, higher blood transfusion rates, and similar hysterectomy rates compared to scheduled repeat CS. The authors concluded that based on the outcomes measured, successful VBAC was associated with the least morbidity, followed by scheduled repeat CS, followed by failed TOLAC with the highest morbidity. The problem, therefore, is that the outcome with the lowest morbidity (successful VBAC) and the procedure with the highest morbidity (failed TOLAC) can both result from the same course of action – the decision to have a TOLAC.

Table 9 summarises the maternal and neonatal risks associated with repeat CS compared to TOLAC. The condition associated with potentially the worst maternal morbidity – uterine rupture – is an uncommon complication and occurs more frequently during TOLAC than during repeat CS. Additionally, while repeat CS appears to decrease the risk of stillbirth, it is important to note that TOLAC does not increase the risk of stillbirth above the baseline risk at any given gestational age. Finally, the described advantages of successful VBAC include avoidance of major abdominal surgery, shorter time to recovery, less morbidity from infection,

Table 9 Comparison of maternal and neonatal risks between repeat CS and TOLAC[24,34]

Maternal risks	Repeat CS (%)	Trial of labour after CS (%)	
		After one CS	After two CSs
Uterine rupture	0.02–0.50	0.70–0.90	0.90–1.80
Hysterectomy	0–0.50	0.10–0.50	0.60
Blood transfusion	0.50–1.40	0.70–1.70	3.20
Endometritis and other infectious morbidity	1.50–3.20	2.90–4.60	3.10
Operative injury	0.30–0.60	0.40–1.30	0.40
Maternal death	0.01–0.04	0.002–0.02	0
Neonatal risks			
Stillbirth			
37–8 weeks	0.08	0.38	
≥39 weeks	0.01	0.16	
Antepartum	0.21	0.10	
Intrapartum	0–0.04	0.01–0.04	
Neonatal death	0.05–0.06	0.08–0.11	
Hypoxic–ischemic encephalopathy	0–0.32	0.08–0.90	
Respiratory morbidity	1.00–5.00	0.10–5.40	
Transient tachypnea	4.20–6.20	3.60	
Hyperbilirubinemia	5.80	2.20	

and avoidance of the increased risk of abnormally invasive placentation in future pregnancies, which is especially important if a large family is desired.

5.2 Magagement Options: Pre-pregnancy and Prenatal

5.2.1 Assessing the Likelihood of a Successful VBAC

Rates of successful VBAC range from 50 to 85%, depending on the reported source. These rates, however, vary depending on several modifiable and/or unmodifiable factors. Strong predictors of a successful VBAC include women with a history of a prior vaginal birth and women who experience spontaneous labour. In contrast, factors that decrease likelihood of success include a recurrence of the indication for the initial caesarean (e.g. arrest of dilatation or descent), gestational age >40 weeks, maternal obesity, pre-eclampsia, short interpregnancy interval, increased maternal age, and non-white ethnicity.

Since the morbidity with failed TOLAC is greater than with successful VBAC, it is useful to assess the likelihood of the women having a successful VBAC. A tool for both women and clinicians when discussing likely success rates may be an online tool (https://mfmunetwork.bsc.gwu.edu/web/mfmunetwork/vaginal-birth-after-caesarean-calculator) that uses many of these variables to calculate an individual's likelihood of successful VBAC.[35,36] Whether such instruments change the decisions made remains unknown as there have been no prospective randomised trials of their use.

5.2.2 Counselling Women

When discussing mode of birth early in pregnancy with women who have had a previous CD, risks (Table 9) and evidence-based recommendations (Table 8) should be addressed. Similarly, it is important to discuss with a patient the strong or poor predictors of success discussed in Section 5.2.1. However, none of these conditions, whether combined or in isolation, is an absolute contraindication to TOLAC if strongly desired by the woman. Autonomy in this regard has to be respected (in many jurisdictions, caesarean section cannot be performed without the woman's consent unless she is judged by a court to be incapable of making a rational decision).[37]

5.3 Management Options: Labour and Delivery

Based on expert consensus, several recommendations regarding labour and delivery have been proposed. These include the location and timing of delivery, operating room availability, and intrapartum management considerations. In general, timing of delivery should be based on routine obstetrical conditions and standards of care. If a repeat CS is planned, this should be scheduled between 39^{+0} weeks and 40^{+0} weeks, unless there is a medical indication to suggest otherwise. Conversely, if a trial of labour is scheduled, success increases substantially if labour commences spontaneously beforehand. Alternatively, induction of labour is not contraindicated in those with a previous CS and may be considered for standard obstetric indications, including postdates pregnancy, provided the woman is fully counselled and accepts the additional risks (and benefits) involved.

If induction of labour is performed, for either maternal or fetal indications prior to spontaneous labour or for postdates, medications that minimise the risk of uterine rupture should be used. In a clinical review of induction methods for women undergoing a trial of labour, Ofir et al. summarised the literature regarding the safest methods of cervical ripening.[38] Of particular importance, prostaglandins such as PGE_1 (misoprostol) and PGE_2 (dinoprostone) deserve special attention. Ofir et al. combined data from seven studies involving 307 women receiving PGE_1 compared to 1,438 women experiencing spontaneous onset of labour, and a more than seven-fold increased odds of uterine rupture was noted in the PGE_1 cohort. Similarly, nine studies involving 3,841 women receiving PGE_2 compared to 32,020 women experiencing spontaneous onset of labour noted 1.7-fold increased odds of uterine rupture in the PGE_2 cohort. These adverse outcomes have led national organisations such as ACOG and SOGC to strongly recommend against the use of these agents in the setting of induction of labour in women with a previous caesarean. Alternatives to prostaglandins that are not contraindicated include mechanical dilatation with a cervical Foley catheter, amniotomy, and judicious use of oxytocin. These should be considered first-line methods of cervical ripening and induction.

Other intrapartum interventions recommended based on expert consensus include continuous fetal monitoring during labour, because up to 70% of uterine rupture cases demonstrate abnormal fetal heart tracings. For example, in a retrospective study of 36 uterine rupture cases, Ridgeway et al. identified a significantly higher rate of fetal bradycardia in the first and second stages of labour compared to 100 controls.[39]

Finally, to facilitate rapid delivery in the setting of suspected uterine rupture, expert consensus recommends that labour should take place in a maternity unit where there is the ability to perform a speedy emergency caesarean. While this recommendation is clearly stated in national guidelines from ACOG, RCOG, and SOGC, there are no described criteria that define exactly what infrastructure is required to meet that objective. In general, 24-hour availability of anaesthesia, operating room support staff, paediatric support, and a provider capable of performing CS is necessary for a centre to offer TOLAC. There is a paucity of data comparing outcomes in women who deliver in different healthcare systems, or in systems with different delivery volumes, thus limiting direct recommendations.

5.4 Secondary/Repeat Caesarean: Summary of Management Options

- Pre-pregnancy and prenatal
  - Discuss mode of delivery with women who have had a previous CD both following that procedure and early in a subsequent pregnancy.
    - Give information in a way that the woman understands, taking into account personal, cultural, and religious factors.
    - Ensure that the woman's view is central to decision-making.
    - Explain the risks (see Table 9).

- Inform her of the evidence-based recommendations (see Table 8).
- Assess the likelihood of a successful VBAC.

- Labour/delivery
  - If TOLAC is chosen
    - this should take place in a setting with immediate access to an operating theatre.
    - continuous fetal heart rate monitoring should be undertaken.
    - Onset of labour:
      - Spontaneous onset of labour is associated with a higher rate of successful vaginal birth than induced labour. Thus, induction should only be considered for standard obstetric indications.
      - Acceptable methods for induction of labour include prudent use of oxytocin, mechanical cervical dilatation with a transcervical balloon, and amniotomy. Prostaglandin methods of cervical ripening may increase the risk of uterine rupture by up to seven-fold if PGE_1 and up to two-fold if PGE_2 is used.
  - If repeat CS is planned
    - this should take place between 39^{+0}–40^{+0} weeks.
    - evidence-based approaches to all aspects of the procedure should be followed (see Table 7).
- Postnatal
  - Care of the baby – this is the same as for a primary CS
  - Care of the woman – this is the same as for a primary CS
  - A discussion about the implications for future pregnancies should be offered (see Table 8).

6 Conclusion

Pregnancy and childbirth expectations and outcomes have changed dramatically over the last 50 years and as CD has become safer, a nuanced discussion of optimal mode of delivery is inevitable and welcomed. Principles of evidence-based practice enables the healthcare professional both to be better informed and to communicate that information to the patient. Caesarean surgical technique is one of the most studied procedures, with over 350 RCTs, meta-analyses, and systematic reviews performed since 1950. When caesarean is indicated and performed, an evidence-based standardised technique may be used to optimise outcomes. Furthermore, when assessing the evidence on the delivery options following a caesarean, a multitude of variables must be synthesised, including institutional policies, maternal and neonatal risks and benefits of each scenario, the implications of each delivery option on future pregnancies, and the desires of the patient in relation to these risks. Ultimately, the goal of thorough counseling and documentation should be a mutually endorsed decision that optimises maternal and neonatal outcomes grounded in the best available evidence.

Further Reading

Robson MS. Can we reduce the caesarean section rate? Best Pract Res Clin Obstet Gynaecol 2001;15:179–94.

Robson MS, Scudamore IW, Walsh SM. Using the medical audit cycle to reduce cesarean section rates. Am J Obstet Gynecol 1996;174:199–205.

Robson M, Murphy M, Byrne F. Quality assurance: the 10-Group Classification System (Robson classification), induction of labor, and cesarean delivery. Int J Gynaecol Obstet 2015;131(S1):S23–7.

Boyle A, Reddy UM, Landy HJ, et al. Primary cesarean delivery in the United States. Obstet Gynecol 2013;122(1):33–40.

Dahlke JD, Mendez-Figueroa H, Rouse DJ, et al. Evidence-based surgery for cesarean delivery: an updated systematic review. Am J Obstet Gynecol 2013; 209(4):294–306.

Dahlke JD, Mendez-Figueroa H, Maggio L, et al. The case for standardizing cesarean delivery technique: seeing the forest for the trees. Obstet Gynecol 2020;136(5):972–80.

Landon MB, Hauth JC, Leveno KJ, et al.; National Institute of Child Health and Human Development Maternal-Fetal Medicine Units Network. Maternal and perinatal outcomes associated with a trial of labor after prior cesarean delivery. N Engl J Med 2004;351:2581–9.

References

1. Centers for Disease Control and Prevention, National Center for Health Statistics. Births: method of delivery. www.cdc.gov/nchs/fastats/delivery .htm (accessed 9 September 2024).

2. National Institute for Health and Care Excellence. Caesarean section. NICE Clinical Guideline. NG192. www.nice.org.uk/guidance/ng192 (accessed 9 September 2024).

3. Zhang Y, Betran AP, Li X, et al. What is an appropriate Caesarean delivery rate for China: a multicentre survey. BJOG 2022;129(1):138–47. http://dx .doi.org/10.1111/1471-0528.16951.

4. Department of Health and Social Care, England. Child and maternal health. https://fingertips.phe.org.uk/profile/child-health-profiles/data#page/1/gid/ 1938133222 (accessed 9 September 2024).

5. Scottish Government. The Best Start – caesarean section rates: review report. www.gov.scot/publications/best-start-review-caesarean-section-rates-scotland/pages/3/ (accessed 1 March 2023).

6. Boerma T, Ronsmans C, Melesse DY, et al. Global epidemiology of use of and disparities in caesarean sections. Lancet 2018;392:1341–8.

7. Hamilton BE, Martin JA, Osterman MJK. Births: provisional data for 2019. Vital Statistics Rapid Release; no 8. www.cdc.gov/nchs/data/vsrr/vsrr-8-508.pdf (accessed 9 September 2024).

8. Zhang J, Troendle J, Reddy UM, et al. Contemporary cesarean delivery practice in the United States. Am J Obstet Gynecol 2010;203:326.e1–10.

9. Healthy People 2030. www.healthypeople.gov (accessed 9 September 2024).

10. McCulloch P, Nagendran M, Campbell WB, et al. Strategies to reduce variation in the use of surgery. Lancet 2013;382:1130–9.

11. Robson MS. Can we reduce the caesarean section rate? Best Pract Res Clin Obstet Gynaecol 2001;15:179–94.

12. Clark SL, Garite TJ, Hamilton EF, Belfort MA, Hankins GD. ''Doing something' about the cesarean delivery rate. Am J Obstet Gynecol. 2018; 219(3):267–71.

13. Stutchfield P, Whitaker R, Russell I. Antenatal betamethasone and incidence of neonatal respiratory distress after elective caesarean section: pragmatic randomised trial. BMJ 2005;331(7518):662. http://dx.doi.org/ 10.1136/bmj.38547.416493.06.

14. Cardwell CR, Stene LC, Joner G, et al. Caesarean section is associated with an increased risk of childhood-onset type 1 diabetes mellitus: a meta-analysis of observational studies. Diabetologia 2008;51:726–35.

15. Thavagnanam S, Fleming J, Bromley A, Shields MD, Cardwell CR. A meta-analysis of the association between caesarean section and childhood asthma. Clin Exp Allergy 2008;38:629–33.

16. Shao Y, Forster SC, Tsaliki E, et al. Stunted microbiota and opportunistic pathogen colonization in caesarean-section birth. Nature 2019;574(7776): 117–121. http://dx.doi.org/10.1038/s41586-019-1560-1.

17. Lurie S, Glezerman M. The history of cesarean technique. Am J Obstet Gynecol 2003;189(6):1803–6, http://dx.doi.org/10.1016/s0002-9378(03) 00856-1.

18. Baskett TF, Calder AA, Arulkamaran S (eds.). Munro Kerr's Operative Obstetrics, 12th edn. London: Saunders, 2014, pp. 132–44.

19. Thaens A, Bonnaerens A, Martens G, et al. Understanding rising caesarean section trends: relevance of inductions and prelabour obstetric interventions at term. Facts Views Vis Obgyn 2011;3:286–91.

20. Robson M, Hartigan L, Murphy M. Methods of achieving and maintaining an appropriate caesarean section rate. Best Pract Res Clin Obstet Gynaecol 2013;27:297–308.

21. Robson M, Murphy M, Byrne F. Quality assurance: the 10-Group Classification System (Robson classification), induction of labor, and cesarean delivery. Int J Gynaecol Obstet 2015;131(S1):S23–7.

22. National Maternity Hospital. Annual Report 2013. Dublin: National Maternity Hospital, 2013. www.lenus.ie/handle/10147/324517 (accessed 9 September 2024).

23. Boyle A, Reddy UM, Landy HJ, et al. Primary cesarean delivery in the United States. Obstet Gynecol 2013;122(1):33–40.

24. Committee on Practice Bulletins-Obstetrics. Practice Bulletin No. 184: Vaginal birth after cesarean delivery. Obstet Gynecol 2017;130:e217–33.

25. American College of Obstetricians and Gynecologists, Society for Maternal-Fetal Medicine; Caughey AB, Cahill AG, Guise JM, Rouse DJ. Obstetric care consensus: safe prevention of the primary cesarean delivery. Am J Obstet Gynecol 2014;210:179–93.

26. Berghella V, Baxter JK, Chauhan SP. Evidence-based surgery for cesarean delivery. Am J Obstet Gynecol 2005;193(5):1607–17.

27. Dahlke JD, Mendez-Figueroa H, Rouse DJ, et al. Evidence-based surgery for cesarean delivery: an updated systematic review. Am J Obstet Gynecol 2013;209(4):294–306.

28. Dahlke JD, Mendez-Figueroa H, Maggio L, et al. The case for standardizing cesarean delivery technique: seeing the forest for the trees. Obstet Gynecol 2020;136(5):972–80.

29. Guyatt GH, Oxman AD, Vist GE, et al. GRADE: an emerging consensus on rating quality of evidence and strength of recommendations. BMJ 2008; 336:924–6.

30. Dodd JM, Crowther CA, Grivell RM, Deussen AR. Elective repeat caesarean section versus induction of labour for women with a previous caesarean birth. Cochrane Database Syst Rev 2017;7(7):CD004906.

31. Royal College of Obstetricians and Gynaecologists (RCOG). Birth after Previous Caesarean Birth. Green-top Guideline No. 45. London: RCOG, 2015. www.rcog.org.uk/globalassets/documents/guidelines/gtg_45.pdf (accessed 9 September 2024).

32. Society of Obstetricians and Gynaecologists of Canada (SOGC). SOGC clinical practice guidelines. Guidelines for vaginal birth after previous caesarean birth. Number 155 (Replaces guideline Number 147), February 2005. Int J Gynaecol Obstet 2005;89(3):319–31.

33. Rossi AC, D'Addario V. Maternal morbidity following a trial of labor after cesarean section vs elective repeat cesarean delivery: a systematic review with metaanalysis. Am J Obstet Gynecol 2008;199:224–31.

34. Hibbard JU, Ismail MA, Wang Y, et al. Failed vaginal birth after a cesarean section: how risky is it? I. Maternal morbidity. Am J Obstet Gynecol 2001;184(7):1365–71; discussion 1371–3.

35. Landon MB, Hauth JC, Leveno KJ, et al.; National Institute of Child Health and Human Development Maternal-Fetal Medicine Units Network. Maternal and perinatal outcomes associated with a trial of labor after prior cesarean delivery. N Engl J Med 2004;351:2581–9.

36. Grobman WA, Sandoval G, Rice MM, et al.; Eunice Kennedy Shriver National Institute of Child Health and Human Development Maternal-Fetal Medicine Units (MFMU) Network. Prediction of vaginal birth after cesarean in term gestations: a calculator without race and ethnicity. Am J Obstet Gynecol 2021;225(6):664.e1–7.

37. Edozien L. Court-authorised caesarean section. BJOG 2014;121(9):1096. http://dx.doi.org/10.1111/1471-0528.12721.

38. Ofir K, Sheiner E, Levy A, Katz M, Mazor M. Uterine rupture: risk factors and pregnancy outcome. Am J Obstet Gynecol 2003;189:1042–6.

39. Ridgeway JJ, Weyrich DL, Benedetti TJ. Fetal heart rate changes associated with uterine rupture. Obstet Gynecol 2004;103:506–12.

High-Risk Pregnancy: Management Options

Professor David James

Emeritus Professor, University of Nottingham, UK

David James was Professor of Fetomaternal Medicine at the University of Nottingham from 1992–2009. The post involved clinical service, especially the management of high-risk pregnancies, guideline development, research and teaching and NHS management. From 2009–14 he was Clinical Director of Women's Health at the National Centre for Clinical Excellence for Women's and Children's Health. He was also Clinical Lead for the RCOG/RCM/eLfH eFM E-Learning Project. He is a recognised authority on the management of problem/complicated pregnancies with over 200 peer-reviewed publications. He has published 16 books, the best-known being *High-Risk Pregnancy: Management Options*.

Professor Philip Steer

Emeritus Professor, Imperial College, London, UK

Philip Steer is Emeritus Professor of Obstetrics at Imperial College London, having been appointed Professor in 1989. He was a consultant obstetrician for 35 years. He was Editor-in-Chief of *BJOG – An International Journal of Obstetrics and Gynaecology* – from 2005–2012, and is now Editor Emeritus. He has published more than 150 peer-reviewed research papers, 109 reviews and editorials and 66 book chapters/books, the best known and most successful being *High-Risk Pregnancy: Management Options*. The fifth edition was published in 2018. He has been President of the British Association of Perinatal Medicine and President of the Section of Obstetrics and Gynaecology of the Royal Society of Medicine. He is an honorary fellow of the College of Obstetricians and Gynecologists of South Africa, and of the American Gynecological & Obstetrical Society.

Professor Carl Weiner

Creighton University School of Medicine, Phoenix, AZ, USA

Carl Weiner is presently Head of Maternal Fetal Medicine for the CommonSpirit Health System, Arizona, Director of Maternal Fetal Medicine, Dignity St Joseph's Hospital, Professor, Obstetrics and Gynecology, Creighton School of Medicine, Phoenix, and Professor, College of Health Solutions, Arizona State University. He is the former Krantz Professor and Chair of Obstetrics and Gynecology, Division Head Maternal Fetal Medicine and Professor Molecular and Integrative Physiology at the University of Kansas School of Medicine, Kansas City, KS and the Crenshaw Professor and Chair of Obstetrics, Gynecology and Reproductive Biology, Division Head Maternal Fetal Medicine, and Professor of Physiology at the University of Maryland School of Medicine, Baltimore. Dr Weiner has published more than 265 peer-reviewed research articles and authored/edited 18 textbooks including *High-Risk Pregnancy: Management Options*. His research was extramurally funded for more than 30 years without interruption.

Professor Stephen Robson

Newcastle University, UK

Stephen C. Robson is Emeritus Professor of Fetal Medicine for the Population and Health Sciences Institute at The Medical School, Newcastle University. He is also a Consultant in Fetal Medicine for Newcastle upon Tyne Hospitals NHS Foundation Trust. He has published over 400 peer-reviewed articles and edited several; books, the highly successful being *High Risk Pregnancy: Management Options*. The fifth edition was published in 2018. He has been President of the British Maternal and Fetal Medicine.

About the Series

Most pregnancies are uncomplicated. However, for some ('high-risk' pregnancies) an adverse outcome for the mother and/or the baby is more likely. Each Element in the series covers a specific high-risk problem/condition in pregnancy. The risks of the condition will be listed followed by an evidence-based review of the management options. Once the series is complete, the Elements will be collated and printed in a sixth edition of *High-Risk Pregnancy: Management Options*.

Cambridge Elements ≡

High-Risk Pregnancy: Management Options

Elements in the Series

Fetal Compromise in Labor
Mark I. Evans, Lawrence D. Devoe and Philip J. Steer

*Spontaneous Preterm Labour and Birth (Including Preterm
Pre-labour Rupture of Membranes)*
Natasha L. Hezelgrave and Andrew H. Shennan

Multiple Pregnancy
Jack Hamer, Jennifer Tamblyn, James Castleman and R. Katie Morris

Diabetes in Pregnancy
Lee Wai Kheong Ryan, Lim Weiying, Ann Margaret Wright and Lay-Kok Tan

Caesarean Section Delivery
Joshua D. Dahlke and Suneet P. Chauhan

A full series listing is available at: www.cambridge.org/EHRP